For all of my teachers and students
big and small.

-MG

KID power Yoga

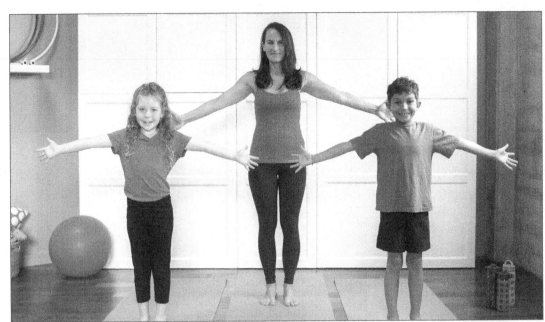

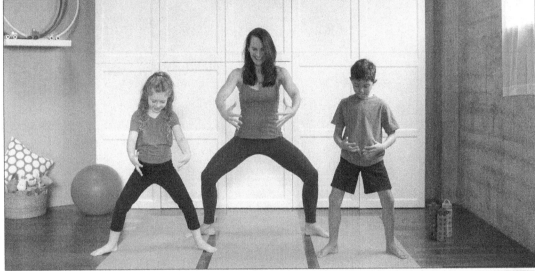

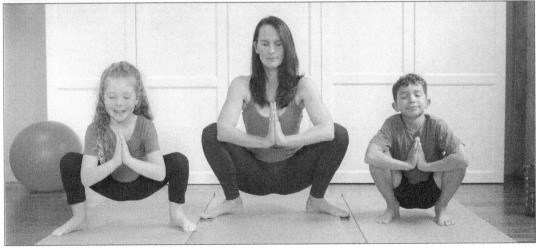

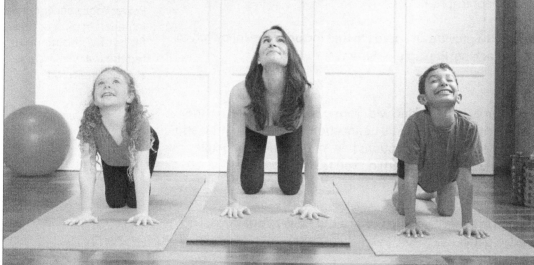

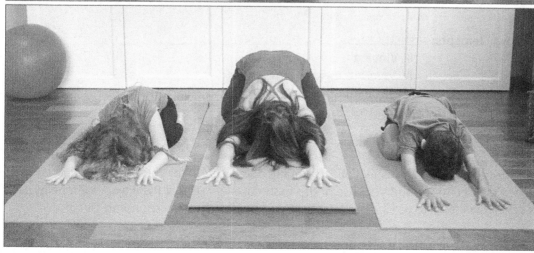

KID power Yoga

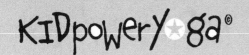

Introduction: How to Use This Manual

———— ★ ————

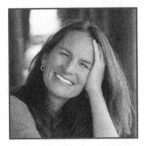

Welcome to the Kid Power Yoga Teacher Training! I am so pleased you are bringing yoga into kids lives. I find that the people who pursue mind/body education and connect to its power in kids' lives are an inspiring and self-selecting group.

Whether you are already doing this work, or have an innate capacity to work with young people, I have no doubt that you will take this training and these materials and use them to express your own creative genius in the world. With that in mind, it is extremely important that this information be of value to you, so let's take a look at how best to use this manual:

The purpose of this training manual is to give you time-tested materials, tools, principles and templates that can be used to create powerful yoga classes and experiences for young people (pre-K-12).

The training is designed to provide an approach that includes the following to support all aspects of teaching: Principle — Structure — Practice.

Principle:

The Kid Power Yoga approach to working with young people is rooted in the **5 Core Principles of Teaching** (Preparation, Connection, Emphasis, Tempo and Self-Study). You will find extensive descriptions here of how these principles can be used to design and improve everything you teach.

Structure:

The next sections detail the specific **Structure of a Kid Power Yoga class.** Each element is outlined and its purpose is described in detail.

Note:

In this manual, you will find guidance and easy steps to follow as well as tools to assess your own growth as a teacher. The idea is to give you fundamental principles and an approach that will enable you to create countless variations and renditions of classes utilizing the specific elements received here.

Every aspect of this training becomes yours in the classroom. If you use Kid Power Yoga concepts and materials in print or other forms of distribution, we require that you ascribe appropriate credit.

— Namasté!

Kid Power Yoga Class Elements:
(Optional: Ritual)
I. Warm Up
II. Building Blocks
III. VInyasa
IV. Savasana/Relaxation
V. Closing Ritual

Practice:

There is a lot of opportunity to take each aspect of the training and try it out for yourself. All of the templates and models have been created to support your use of this material every step of the way. Additionally, each class section also offers specific material to use in your classes (supported by the corresponding DVD).

Let's get started!

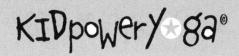

Table of Contents

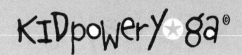

I. Quick Preview—Putting the work into action!

Here are the easy 5 Easy Steps to Creating an Effective Kid Power Yoga Class:

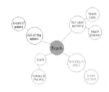

1. Mind Map (pg 67) Choose a theme, start anywhere and let your ideas flow. Let yourself think outside of the box here and just see what comes out.

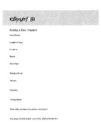

2. Use the KPY Template (pg 76) to write out your class. Pay attention to how you will start your class (ritual + warm up) your transitions, which poses do you want to specifically teach (building blocks), are you using a story based vinyasa or more of a free flow and what is your intention in doing that? What will you use for your relaxation/calm rest (savasana) at the end of the class? Will there be a closing ritual? *(Review the 5 Core Principles of Teaching pg 10)*

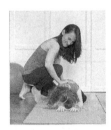

3. Teach the Class! Teach to your own children, an existing class, teach your nephew, teach your spouse, teach your best friend… just teach!

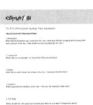

4. Assess the Class (using the 5 Core Principles of Teaching: Class Assessment pg 78)

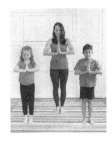

5. Teach Again *(See below)*

To Grow as a Teacher You Have to Teach

Your goal for your Kid Power Yoga Training may be to work primarily with your own children or in a classroom. Either way, to grow as a teacher you have to teach.

If you do not have children to teach and you want to continue on this path, go ahead and create opportunities for yourself.

Notes:

_____

_____

_____

_____

_____

_____

_____

_____

_____

_____

_____

_____

_____

_____

_____

_____

_____

_____

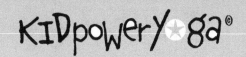

II. Vinyasa Yoga and Kids—Why Flow?

Asana (a yoga pose) is a form of guided meditation using the body and the breath to anchor one's attention in the present moment. This is as true for young people as it is for adults.

Vinyasa (meaning 'flow') is a style of yoga that uses fluid movement, as opposed to static holdings as the means for accessing the powerful benefits that yoga has to offer. Vinyasa taps into that part of human experience that responds to song, to dance, to poetry. It is about rhythm, stillness and a uniquely playful way of moving the body through the ancient practice of yoga.

We would like to believe that young people have a healthy range of motion and strength, but the truth is that ability levels in kids are as varied as they are in adults. Vinyasa allows for many different points of entry into the practice for young people because of its fluid shifting from one posture to the next. For instance, if a student is less skilled in balance, she has the opportunity to practice it in one moment, and then move into another posture that may simply require a straight arm and bent knee. She can practice in areas that require improvement while staying calm and easy-going under minor stress, then flow into a posture that gives her a sense of success again.

The easy movement from one posture to the next also increases coordination and can be learned almost like a dance or martial arts sequence through specific flow sequences (like Sun Salutations pg 55). The emphasis on movement in Vinyasa also increases cardiovascular benefits because students will use their entire bodies throughout a class, flowing through multiple postures, accessing all lines of the body.

In terms of engagement, Vinyasa's inherent 'flow' is a perfect vehicle for story-telling, creativity and yoga 'games.' The Vinyasa class serves as an ideal canvas for an Instructor's inspiration and creativity to play out within the structure/container of the class.

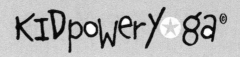

Notes:

_____

_____

_____

_____

_____

_____

_____

_____

_____

_____

_____

_____

_____

_____

_____

_____

_____

_____

_____

_____

_____

_____

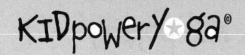

III. The 5 Core Principles of Teaching – The Through-Line of the KPY Program

These principles below are the through line for the Kid Power Yoga program. These key elements can be used to help structure and assess any class.

1. Preparation:

"Luck is what happens when preparation meets opportunity."
–Lucius Annaeus Seneca

Preparation is a key ingredient for success. Any teacher of any subject knows firsthand the power of good preparation and the pitfalls of being without it.

Note:

Of course there is a level of forgiveness in any class if your music malfunctions or your phone starts ringing and part of teaching yoga is modeling literally how to 'go with the flow.' One can always recover. But, overall, your preparation will make an enormous difference in how comfortable you feel and how well you can focus on the actual experience you wish to create.

This is not to say that everything must go as planned to be successful.
Some of the best classes have a spark of inspiration halfway through that may shift the course in an exciting way. But we cannot be available to respond to those spontaneous shifts or receive divine inspiration if we are struggling to salvage a class from a lack of preparation. We simply won't see the opportunity.

Preparation of Self includes:
- Knowing what you are going to teach that day.
- Having visual cues to remain on track, such as written templates and class cards.
- Keeping materials/props ready and accessible. (If you have to get up to go get something out of your bag several times during the class it can throw off the connection and tempo.)
- Having music already cued.
- Turning phones off.

(Also see: Rituals pg 22)

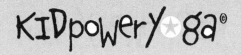

Preparation Questions Guide:
What do I need to prepare myself to teach?
How should I prepare my classes?
What type of support do students need to participate?

Preparation In Action:
I recently taught yoga to a 5th grade class. I only get to see them once a month because of all of the standard requirements in higher elementary grade levels, so I often feel a bit like I am 'starting from scratch' each time I teach this group. I promised them that we would enjoy a class outside when the weather changed. Finally it arrived, a gorgeous day with blue sky and sunshine. Knowing that I was about to unleash twenty-eight 10 year-olds onto an open field for a very 'out of their element' experience, I had to make sure my physical preparation of the space was impeccable. I set up every one of those 28 yoga mats in a large circle with myself in the center. By the time they came outside, I was sitting down with my shoes placed neatly behind my mat, waiting for them as peacefully as possible. I used minimal gestures and almost no language to show them what was expected, keeping myself as quiet as possible. They followed suit, not because they are a particularly mellow group, but because it was a novelty and the environment was well prepared. They were receptive to clear instruction about where to go and what to do next. Without that, I am fairly certain I'd still be on that field chasing them to set up their yoga mats.

2. Connection:

"To the world you may be just one person, but to one person you may be the world." –Brandi Snyder

Connection in a class is essential. This includes connection to the material you are teaching as well as to the students.

Connection to the Material:
Finding connection with the material should not be too difficult to achieve because you will be choosing the themes and the emphasis within the yoga classes.

However, since you will be using new tools from this program, 'trying them on' to see how they fit, have some patience with the process. If you discover ways to make something more your own, please to do so.

Note: Many people teach the elements of this course exactly as they are given and never change a thing. If you are newer to working with young people, you may not yet be able to discern what feels most comfortable and feels most like 'you'. In that case, try everything as it is laid out and see how it unfolds. You will naturally learn how to make adjustments. The mind-mapping strategies also allow for great creativity.

I had a Teacher Training student who did not connect to the image of resting on a cloud and sailing into the sky (Relaxation Techniques/ Guided Meditation). He chose ultimately to work with the image of a boat. He grew up with boats and had wonderful memories of sailing with his Dad. For him, a boat gently rocking and journeying to new worlds was a potent image and something he felt he could communicate well. I have no doubt that the more powerful choice for him was to use that image and that trying to give a guided meditation to kids about being in the clouds would have felt less authentic for his students.

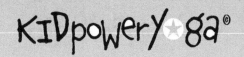

Look for the images, ideas and directions you feel most drawn to intuitively. Ultimately, having a passion for what you teach will translate to students.

Connection to Students:
This will also come very naturally. Kids' Yoga Teachers are a self-selecting group and young people are a very compelling audience. However, you may come across a student who you do not feel a connection with or who you may not find particularly enjoyable. This is normal and ultimately presents a great opportunity. This situation requires finding ways to engage differently (possibly by asking him/her for specific feedback). It also requires personal reflection to learn why this child is more challenging for you than others (See Self Study).

Connection Questions Guide:
How am I connecting to the kids in this room?
How connected do they feel to what I am teaching?
How connected do I feel to what I am teaching?
Where can my awareness and 'connection' support what I am teaching?

Connection in Action:
A few years ago, a school district invited me to work with their entire 4th grade community. It was an initiative designed to support 'anti-stress' techniques during the standardized testing season. I was teaching four different 4th grade classes in a row, once a week. The class was held inside of a large gym and I prepared my mats in a circle before the students arrived. They would file in, choose a mat, take class, and then file out of the gym, passing the next line of kids waiting for class. After the first week, the names and faces became a blur. After the second week, I could see that the newness of the experience was wearing off and that I needed to create more connection with each group if we were going to gel together. I was running the risk of being more like an assembly than a place for them to learn new relaxation tools. I realized I was overlooking the most obvious thing; I did not know their names! I would not be there all year, so I wasn't even really trying to know them individually. It is hard to feel like someone is taking an interest in you if they do not take the time to learn your name. So, I made sure I did. I began creating a class roster and organized a 'mat chart'. By the end of the next session, I had almost all of them identified. It made a difference. They responded differently to me when I was able to greet them by name as he or she came in the room. And not surprisingly, the classes went more smoothly and we created a set of testing tools the school still uses today.

When starting out, it can be challenging deciding whether to match the energy in the room or to change it. When I began teaching, if the students entered the room and seemed very boisterous, I might shift my plan to get them to calm down with a very mellow and relaxing warm up. I learned over time that the wilder energy just needs to express itself and I became less afraid of stirring them up with a more active warm up to better meet their energy level. The best way to learn tempo is through practice.

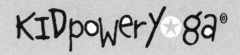

3. Tempo

"Music is the space between the notes." –Claude Debussy

Tempo can be one of the biggest challenges to new instructors. The more you teach, the easier it becomes to intuit the best pace or rhythm in a given class, allowing for periods of higher energy and moments of stillness.

When creating a class, the one part we cannot completely anticipate is the students themselves; their questions, responses, likes, dislikes, focus and silliness on a given day has an enormous effect on how the class flows. Tempo is the way in which we, as conductors, take the previously orchestrated class structure and weave it together with the actual performances in front of us to create a beautiful symphony.

When I first began teaching, I constantly had one of two experiences:
I. It took forever to get through something I thought would be a quick 'go around the room' question to the students.
II. I would finish the entire class 10 minutes before I intended and be left with either trying to extend savasana (not possible after a while) or scrambling to think of one more activity. (See Preparation: Always have a few more things planned than you may finish.)

Tempo Questions Guide: What is the tempo of my classes?
• Do I allow for both calm and active energies or do I teach at only one pace?
• Where and how can I make helpful shifts?
• What is the tempo of each section of my class and what are my transitions?

Tempo in Action: Tempo is so much about intuition and in my experience, what we think of as 'intuition' is often the result of a lot of experience. All that is to say, tempo gets easier the longer and more often you teach. I teach a weekly kindergarten class that meets just after lunch. This is a bit of a challenge because they have been moving, a lot, and come in full of recess energy. It is a noisy class in the beginning as kids come in (someone is always late) and shove lunches and coats away and do a 'slide into home plate' to get to their spot on the rug. There are times when I teach that class very quietly, I focus on stillness and breathing, on noticing sensation in the body and simple movements (not as much balancing as they are still a bit in 'silly' mode and will do more crashing to the ground than anything else). Sometimes, we start very slowly and gently.

Emphasis in a class can be an overarching desire to teach kids to have more available responses to adversity. The whole emphasis of what you teach can be how to sit with discomfort or challenges and 'stay in the pose.' That could be a gift to young people in your life that you continue to teach them each week for years.

Emphasis in a given pose could be focused on the experience of the feet and how the four corners press evenly into the earth. Remember, less is more, we are teaching them, yes, but there is no rush, this is a life-long practice and so we give them specific tools to use so they actually have the experience rather than rushing through a lot of instruction.

Emphasis can be contained within a theme you choose for a class. (A theme can be 'the spine' or 'courage' or 'the ocean') but it becomes important as a way to direct your teaching and thereby your students to pay attention to what you specifically want them to get out of the experience.

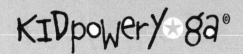

But there are other times, after our regular ritual to transition, that I will let the energy remain big. I have us doing lots of large movements (and sometimes loud stomping and clapping) because it can feel wonderful to share that much energy with a big group. What seems most important is that I am willing to create variations, nothing is always quiet and nothing is always boisterous and engaging. What I want is to create a feeling of community and unity in the room whether we are going very big and loud or still and contemplative. As a teacher, I feel comfortable transitioning through these different energetic states and can flow through them as needed by each class.

4. Emphasis

"In the long run, you only hit what you aim at." –Henry David Thoreau

Emphasis is about intention. This is how you, as a teacher, will reach your students; by teaching through emphasis and personal example.

In teaching, less is more. Even though we may have so much we want students to get out of a pose or an experience, the more focused we are on the essence of what we are teaching, the more clearly they will experience it.

Emphasis Questions Guide:
- What is my emphasis in this class?
- What supports that emphasis and how does that emphasis support my students?
- What am I teaching them today?

Emphasis in Action:
I work with a 3rd grade class weekly and I knew that I wanted to emphasize (for the whole year) the beauty that is available when we get very still and quiet. I wanted to bring more silence into what are often quite lively classes with that age group. Now, I obviously could have talked about silence, and peace and listening inward, and I do cover those topics. But more importantly, I started a mini-flow at the beginning of each session that is entirely silent. We started this method in September, and by May there was no confusion; the beginning of class is a silent yoga practice. That became our first warm up and our ritual. I love that part of the class, the easy way that breath and movement can synchronize when the room is quiet and the only focus in on the yoga. There is an ease and a competence in the gentle movements from upward dog, to the relief of child pose and back again. The room is quietly moving together and there is beauty there. Then, we move into a more active warm up, building blocks, vinyasa (these kids love story-based vinyasa) and finally relaxation. These 8 year-olds are not just being told about silence, or told to be quiet, they are experiencing quiet; they are being silence.

Note:

In the appendix (pg 66) you will find a copy of your own self-assessment template of the *Five Core Principles of Teaching*.

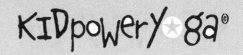

5. Self Study

"We can only teach who we are." –Unknown

As teachers, we can only teach who we are. To grow as a yoga teacher is to grow as a person. Working with young people is an amazing laboratory for self-study. What comes easily to us in teaching, and what throws us for a loop, reveals great information about who we are as individuals.

This training is also a Self Study practice. We take on something like this seeking new ways to expand and grow. The strongest teaching comes from what we demonstrate rather than what we say. Working with young people is 'being the change' 101 and happily it never ends.

Self Study Questions Guide:
- Where am I on this journey?
- What do I need to fill my own cup?
- What else can I learn?
- How can I continue a process that will teach me more about who I am so I can bring more understanding to the young people I work with?

Self Study in Action:
A year ago, I was in a Kindergarten class taught by a very dedicated and beloved classroom teacher. She has over 25 years of experience and is as gifted an educator as I have ever seen. I was coming through to borrow her CD player for my next class and she happened to have a movement break. She is not a yoga teacher, but when she told the kids it was time for the movement break, they easily moved into a large circle and began a focused flow of what was, more or less, sun salutations A + B. Now, I have taught some Kindergartners, but I would not have thought this group was capable of what they were so effortlessly doing in that brief break. It took me by surprise. What was I not asking of the kids I work with? How have I been underestimating what they can do and where we go together? I needed to examine my desire for students to 'love it' and perhaps sacrifice some of what I know

Note:

Themes should only be expansive and helpful and never limiting. If there is something you want to bring into a class, but are not sure how it fits into the "Ocean" theme you have created for example; trust that you can do a foot warm up and then move the students back into your water theme with no problem.

to be the gifts of this practice. That is a fine line, but I also know (and knew in that moment) that I have to always be asking myself the question: Am I afraid of failing and therefore not asking my students to find their best selves? This led me to the silent practice in the 3rd grade class the following year. This is Self Study.

In Conclusion:
The 5 Core Principles of Teaching (Preparation, Connection, Tempo, Emphasis and Self Study) are a diagnostic tool. If something is going well in one of your classes, or not so well, a clear assessment of the 5 Core Principles will allow you to better understand what is happening and what needs (or does not need) to shift.

15

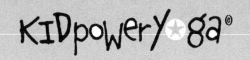

Notes:

KIDpowerYoga®

Notes:

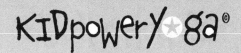

IV. The Use of a Theme in a Kid Power Yoga Class

Theme:

Class Elements:

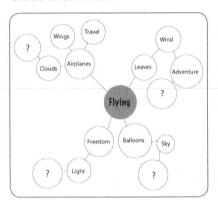

Having a theme for a specific class or class series is very helpful for organizing and articulating intentions for students. Themes can serve as great guides and help support what you want to emphasize in your teaching.

A theme can be overt: A Day at the Beach, Finding Balance in Our Bodies and Our Lives, Healthy Spines

A theme can be subtle: Strength, Letting Go, The Heart

Themes as Organizing Tools: A Mind Map is a way to get started with class planning. The idea is to pick an organizing idea (like Beach pg 67 or Flying) and then just let your creativity flow. It can be amazing to see what can happen when thoughts aren't censored. Those ideas, images, poses will create the basis for future classes. (See Mind Maps to get started pg 70)

Themes as Teaching Tools: Themes allow you to make choices and to organize ideas, which can be a challenge for newer teachers. Themes help to build our classes on both a literal and an energetic level. If we know where we are going and what our emphasis is, we can allow different rhythms and different tempos within our classes. If we are less certain, then that confusion tends to make our classes one dimensional because we are using only our personality to keep a connection with the class and to propel the material forward.

Note: Things to Consider with Rituals
In a perfect world, you are teaching in a dedicated space that is empty before you begin class. In that case, you can set the music, the room, and the activities exactly as you wish. In many other cases, you are teaching in a school or a community center with limited space and kids arrive at the same moment the room is available. Rituals are listed as optional because your 'ritual' may be the warm up or your 'ritual' may be moving desks out of the way, etc. Flexibility is key.

Note on Art Activity Rituals:
If you are doing an art activity, keep in mind that unless it happens within your designated class time, some students will arrive on time or even be late and miss it. For this reason, the art activity has to be something that has meaning, but is also optional. I have made the mistake of having students draw 'drishti' points on sticky notes to focus on during balancing postures and then not had a plan for the students who didn't have one because they arrived late. If you are going to incorporate the 'mini-art' experience into your class, just be sure to have a plan for students who don't participate in the mini-art.

Final Note on Rituals:
Rituals help transitions and clarify intentions but they also allow for increased ownership in the experience as a whole. The more students can anticipate and be involved, the more connected they feel to the experience. They may even begin on their own to learn how to place their shoes, turn on the lights, start spreading mats etc. I was teaching for several months in our studio before I realized that the girls in class were all starting to show up with their hair in the same very messy, quick pull back knot I was throwing my hair into before class. They are paying attention. The more we can do to support them in being connected and take ownership of the experience, the better.

Notes:

_____

_____

_____

_____

_____

_____

_____

_____

_____

_____

_____

_____

_____

_____

_____

_____

_____

_____

_____

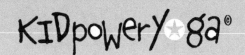

V. The Structure of a Kid Power Yoga Class

Class Elements

Class Elements:
(Optional: Ritual)

V. Warm Up
VI. Building Blocks
VII. VInyasa
VIII. Savasana/Relaxation
IX. Closing Ritual

Ritual (Optional):

A ritual is a way for students to transition from their day into your class. It is a cue that something has shifted and this is now a different, intentional time.

A ritual can be elaborate such as an art activity done in the foyer of a yoga studio that relates to the theme for the class. (Note, if you are doing a pre-class activity such as that, it needs to not be essential to the class as not all students will get there in time to participate. See below.)

The music you played before the start of class can be a form of transition and cue. In many adult studios, the use of a focal cue sends a memory message to the senses that connects to a state of relaxation experienced at the end of a class.

The way students remove and place their shoes can be an effective ritual. (This can be taught in your first classes as an expression of the care and attention students will have in their poses). Each moment brings an opportunity.

Examples of rituals:
- Art activities
- Music to prompt the start of class
- Laying down mats (it can be helpful to already have this set up, but can also be a good ritual; another opportunity to take time and demonstrate care).
- An initial easy flow of postures (can be used as a warm-up, a familiar seated flow can be a great transition and a mini-series the students eventually know by heart).

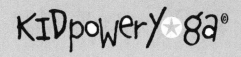

Notes:

_____

_____

_____

_____

_____

_____

_____

_____

_____

_____

_____

_____

_____

_____

_____

_____

_____

_____

_____

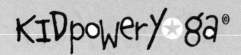

VI. Warm Ups (& Rituals)

In a typical adult Vinyasa class, the Sun Salutations (A + B) are used to support a physical warming of the muscles and lines of the body for upcoming postures. The repetition also serves to move the student out of her head and into her body; out of the day she had and into the present moment of her practice. Similarly, the purpose of a warm up in a Kid Power Yoga class is as much mental and emotional as it is physical.

The warm up in a Kid Power Yoga class is a key component for connection to the students. In all my years of teaching, I've observed that if young people feel engaged in the warm up, they will move into yoga postures and flow bringing all of the focus and attention I could hope for into learning the actual poses. They do need to feel that connection; that this practice is for them. The warm up is a way to bring the yoga to them rather than creating the impression they have to take so many steps to meet the experience.

Some of the warm ups in our repertoire are asana-based, but many of them have a different emphasis. All of them are a communication to the student that says, "I understand that you are kids and ultimately yoga is about joy in your body and in yourself, so let's begin there."

Warm Ups

Rhythms: (Video)
The use of rhythms to focus, calm or transition a group is an age-old classroom teacher tool. It is far more effective than saying 'Ok, ok, we are going to get started… shhhhh.' It is important to 'head out' and let them follow.

Welcome Rhythms:
Rhythms can be incorporated into a name game/way to get to know new kids:
Floor Floor (Hit the floor 2x)
Knee Knee (Hit your knees 2x)

Shoulder Shoulder (Hit your shoulders 2x)
Arms in the air—WELCOME DYLAN!
The whole group can do this by first learning the rhythm and then adding the names. You can vary it by going very fast, very slow, quiet and then loud etc.

Crazy Cookies: (Video)
Follow along Warm Up that encourages participation and tactile awareness. You can expand on crazy cookies by giving anatomical names for the body parts or bones being used.

Yoga Ball:
With the large yoga ball try passing it from one student to another across the circle. Call out specific body part to use—'One finger only, foot only, elbows only, head only etc.' This has the potential to make kids get off their mats and bang into each other so the rules of 'staying on your mat' have to be very clear. Great de-brief is to get their feedback on what was harder and what was easier and discuss how we are used to using our bodies in certain ways but that it is exciting to look at expanding that. (In a bigger way, yoga helps us to use more of our bodies in more ways—increasing our strength and health). Music is a great addition to this warm up.

Beach Ball Toss:
Stand in a circle with the group. Toss a beach ball from one person to another around and across the circle. You can create 'challenges' such seeing how many taps the group can get before it hits the floor This is a good opportunity to explicitly model what support and teamwork looks like with encouraging phrases as people both hit and miss the ball.

Shakey: (Video)
Any kind of movement fun that gets them focused and moving early on is a great way to get engagement. This one is far better understood by watching the DVD.

Balloons: (Video)
This warm up expands on the Yoga Ball and gives each student the opportunity to try the same exercise with their own balloon and different body parts. Music is a great addition to this warm up.

Toe Warm Ups + Tippy Toes: (Video)
Combination of self-massage, body awareness and playful warm up. In this warm up it is important to focus on simple before challenging. Lifting of the big toe before trying to lift the little toe for example keeps students engaged with the experience of 'I can do this!' and then the more

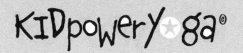

challenging elements are just fun to try. If students have too many experiences in a row of things that are not accessible, engagement will quickly disappear. Music is a great addition to this warm up.

Downward Dog Walk:
Crab Walk (Table Pose) You can add a little 'pinch of the toes' Inch Worm (Flat on the earth, try to lift your bottom and wriggle—is challenging and funny) Snake (Slither across the floor) Music is a great addition to this warm up.

Self Massage/Untying the Knots:
Guiding students in self massage of the neck and shoulder area as though they were untying knots is a great way to promote and teach self-soothing techniques.

Pipe Cleaners: (Teaching about the spine)
First have students find their spines, ribs—feel around for body awareness. Then bring out pipe cleaners—first demonstrating a more or less healthy curvature of the spine. (Of course this can be supplemented with skeletal models). Ask the students to create healthy or unhealthy spines. They will twist the pipe cleaners into incredible loops that is fun for them. Then you can ask them to help make that spine more healthy again. Kids like the experience and the humor of this exercise. It is used to build body awareness.

Warm Ups with Theme:
You can create a warm up with a theme—such as "Things in a Garden." This can include yoga and non-yoga/created poses either led by you or generated by the students or a combination. Once the movements have been learned, you can simply call them out and have the students move into their own embodiment of the 'garden'. (It is helpful if you are creating a warm up like this to have a 'baseline' movement such as wind blowing (swaying arms with swishing noise) to go back to between other poses).

Note: This can also serve as a combo with your building blocks if you want to accomplish both together. Music is a great addition to this warm up.

Om/Namasté (Game):
Like red light/green light
One student is at one end of the room (or you take that role) and says 'oooooooo hhhhhhhhh mmmmmmmm' as students advance toward you. When you wish, you turn and say 'Namasté' and students have to either:
(This part is up to you in terms of the best fit for your class)
-Freeze
-Freeze with hands in Namasté
-Freeze with hands in Namasté in a balancing posture

Crazy Walks:
This series of walks must first be taught to the class and then is a very fun way to allow for play and a very physical warm up at the beginning of your class.

Freeze Dance:
The classic dance and freeze warm up is a lot of fun for students. I begin with students as a pot of water on the stove (curled up in child's pose) and they begin to move as they hear the music until at the boiling point they are completely moving and dancing on their mats/or in their area. When the music stops they freeze and then a volunteer calls out a hot place and they begin moving again. At the end, we all melt slowly down to the ground to a seated position. Music is essential to this warm up.

Sometimes: (Video)
Follow along Warm Up that encourages participation.

Create a Warm Up!
Let a student show a movement to warm up the:
Feet - then everyone does it together
Legs - then everyone does it together
Hips - then everyone does it together
Arms - then everyone does it together
Hands + Fingers...
Neck...
Head (even face)...

This can be done calmly and methodically or with lots of energy and music depending on what you want for the class.

I Know an Old Lady…
Acting out a mini-flow with postures to the song 'I Know an Old Lady Who Swallowed a Fly." (I change the refrain to: 'I know an Old Lady Who Swallowed a Fly—but she did yoga so she felt gooood.'
And 'My oh my' instead of 'I guess she'll die'
Fly pose—can be created by students
Spider
Bird
Cat
Dog
Cow (1/2 of cat tilts or cow pose)
Horse

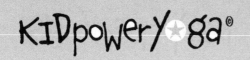

Notes:

_____

_____

_____

_____

_____

_____

_____

_____

_____

_____

_____

_____

_____

_____

_____

_____

_____

_____

_____

KIDpowerYoga©

Notes:

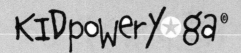

VII. Building Blocks

This 2nd element of a Kid Power Yoga Class introduces specific postures that students will do in the Vinyasa/Flow section of the class. The idea is that at this point your students have become engaged through the warm up and are ready to move into specific instruction.

You do not need to teach every posture in your flow during the building block section of class. Keep in mind, less is more. Teach the concepts you will be going back to and use the building blocks section to work on emphasis.

There are 2 separate things to consider when teaching Building Blocks:

1. How to introduce the pose
2. How to teach the alignment of the pose

How to Introduce the Poses:

Approaches to Introducing Poses:

Follow me	*Workshop*	*Creative*	*Re-teach*
This is a fine default when you want to have students try and learn something without taking a lot of extra time in the presentation. Simply modeling in front of them and having them experiment works well. (With a more experienced group, most of the building blocks may be simply Follow Me because the goal is to get through the instruction, give them the tools and get into the flow section of your class.)	Have one student come up to the front of the room and walk the student through the intended pose first. If it is a review, students can use the alignment tools they already know to be sure that the student who is modeling the pose is focused on the relevant cues 'where are my feet?', 'where are my hands?', 'Where is my gaze?' 'Am I balancing in the pose?' Then everyone else tries it too. This method a very effective way to teach and uses the 'top of the educational triangle' adage, "if I can teach it, I know it".	You can engage students in a myriad of ways: • Pulling postures from a net (Video). • Giving them popsicle sticks with the name of their pose and then having them help teach/lead it. • Giving small groups letters that spell out a posture. Once they figure it out, they come back to the group and everyone learns the posture together.	To reinforce alignment points, it can be helpful to have a student in the middle of the room doing a pose that has been taught and then have the rest of the class run through the key alignment points to ensure that everything is strong.

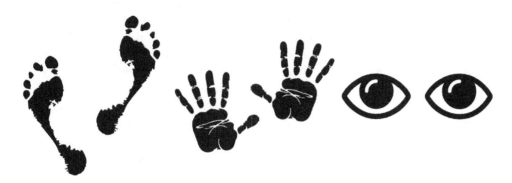

How to Teach the Poses:

Key Alignment Points:

Feet   Hands   Eyes

Depending on age and ability/experience level of developing students, you can bring in more alignment points within a pose. But, from a teaching perspective, keep in mind that you want them to move into the pose and have a personal experience with it. They will experience the pose, if you focus on:

Feet: Where are my feet? Am I pressing them into the earth?

Hands: Where are my hands? Are they awake and alive?

Eyes: Where is my gaze?

Using these three points will bring them 90% of the way to most postures safely. A final helpful question can then be: Am I bringing a balance of focus and calm/ease to the pose? Remember: This is not so different from teaching a beginning level adult class. Keep it Simple.

———★———

Note:
Obviously, anytime students are assessing each other, positive feedback and reinforcement are key. It is then your job as the teacher to help guide the students by making sure they have the key rubric for assessment. (They should already be very clear in the language of Feet/Hands/Eyes) By in large, most students like to 'be the one' in the middle and self-select it so they are comfortable with being 'helped more fully/deeply into the pose by the students' comments. As the teacher, you are also giving positive comments to the student model throughout as they make good adjustments. The 'top of the learning triangle' is to teach back, so the re-teach is a very effective tool.

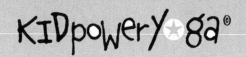

Key Concepts for Safety and Fun:

If it hurts, it is not yoga

There are forms of yoga that work the pain/sensation threshold but that is not appropriate for working with young people. The goal here is awareness, not pushing through pain. Teach them to modify, modify, modify and back off to the point where they can do the pose without discomfort. For some, that will mean a very small amount of movement (see Celebrating Where We Are).

This is not a race

This is a good lesson for us all. There is no competition here. The beauty is that yoga is self-paced and self-reflective. This is what so many kids (and parents) love about the practice.

Celebrating where we are

It is important to explicitly teach students to work from where they are physically. This has to be demonstrated in everything you do. You have to constantly be modeling finding the place that is 'yoga' in each posture, for each individual student. For instance, if a student is overweight, wearing jeans and cannot bring her hands out in front of her or move comfortably - where is her yoga? Anywhere is a beginning and a great place to start. If she can breathe and stay in just that moment and notice anything about the experience, then it's perfect in that moment. Encourage her to take deep breaths and feel the sensation. That is yoga.

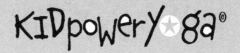

Asana:

Standing Poses:

Mountain (Video):
Feet are pressing into the earth. Spine is long. Shoulders are relaxed. Heart open. Eyes at once point. Hands are at your sides, awake and alive.

Half Moon (Video):
Mountain pose. Bring right hand to your waist, left hand high. Reach with your left hand to your right. Reverse sides.

Gorilla:
Mountain pose. Lean forward. Hands are on your thighs, knees or shins depending on what is comfortable. Extend your spine. Lift one foot and then the other if you wish (more active).

Warrior I (Video):
Step one foot back. Back foot is angled out. Front knee is bent (over the ankle or back—not in front of the ankle). Back leg is straight but not locked. Reach arms overhead.

Warrior II (Video):
Warrior I; Turn your body to the side and reach arm out wide. Front knee is bent. Back leg is straight but not locked. Look out over your fingertips.

Ostrich:
Stand with your legs apart. Hands on your hips and bend forward. Bring hands to the floor if possible or keep at your hips.

Horse (Video):
Stand with your feet apart wide. Knees bent, toes to the sides of your mat. Hands are together at your heart in Namasté. Forearms create a straight line. Shoulders roll back. Heart is open and lifting.

Triangle:
Turn your body to the side and step one foot back and keep one foot forward facing front. Back foot is angled diagonally toward the front corner of the mat. Arms are out to the side as in Warrior II. Bend forward to the side and place your lower hand on your thigh, lightly on the knee or ankle. Upper arm is reaching high. Gaze up at the upper thumbnail.

Bent Knee Triangle:
Bend the front knee just in line with the ankle and follow the steps for Triangle.

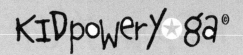

Star:
Feet are stretched out wide. Toes pointing out diagonally. Hands are outstretched to the sides. Take up a lot of space. (Optional: Twinkle by wiggling your fingers)

Wish on a Star (Used more for focus) (Video):
Bring the palms together over your head. Bring them down (hands pressing together) in front of your chest. (Fingers are pointing away from you). Fold the backs of the hands together and continue pressing as you bend your elbows, fold your fingers down and toward you to brush your chest. Then bring your cupped palms to your mouth to 'blow' a wish.

Balancing Poses:

Eagle:
Bring arms out to the sides. Bend your knees, cross right leg over the left. Bend the elbows and bring right arm under the left. Spine is straight. Squat lower. Gaze is at one point. (Optional: Bend Forward)

Tree (Video):
Stand in mountain. Bring your hands to your heart in Namasté. Gaze at one point—eyes are still. Lift one foot and place it on your opposite leg, sole pressing into the standing leg. (Placement can be high—upper thigh, or low—ankle). Repeat on the other side.

Airplane/Bird (Video):
Stand in mountain with your hands at your heart. Gently spread your arms back on each side like wings. Lean forward slightly keeping your heart lifted and bring the back foot off the ground. Eyes are still at one point. Repeat on the other side.

Backbends:

Cobra (Video):
Lying on your belly. Bring your forearms to the floor and lift your head. Continue the length through your spine.

Upward Dog:
From Cobra, bring your hands under your shoulders and press your head and chest up using your arms. Heart is open.

Shark (Video):
Lie on your belly and bring your toes together for your tale. Reach your hands behind your back and clasp—lifting them as a fin—Dun dun dun dun…

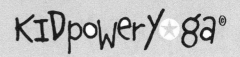

Bridge:

Lie on your back, knees bent and feet hip width apart pressing into the earth. Press your hips up and toward the ceiling, arms can be by your sides or clasping underneath your back.

Inversions:

Candlestick:

Lying on your back, lift your legs straight up into the air. More advanced students may wish to lift the hips supporting their lower back with their hands. Students who find the basic pose challenging, may wish to do it against a wall. (Rear-end and the backs of the legs are then up against the wall for this pose).

Arm-strengthening Poses:

Plank:

Come into the top of a push up. Hands under shoulders, toes tucked. Get very long.

Rainbow (Side plank):

Come into plank and then turn onto your side. Resting on your bottom arm and side edge of the bottom foot. It can be helpful to drop the lower knee to the floor.

Downward Dog (also an inversion) (Video):

Spread your hands and feet onto the floor in an upside down 'V' Hips reach up to the sky. Arms and legs are as straight as possible. Hands are pressing evenly into the earth.

Dolphin:

Come into Downward Dog and then bring your forearms to the floor and rest of them with your hands clasped together.

Table:

Sitting on your bottom, bring your hands behind you, plant your feet into the earth and lift your hips and chest high—Creating a table top with your body.

Seated Poses:

Cat tilts (Video):

Move onto your hands and knees. (Hands under shoulders, knees under hips). Let your belly sink toward the floor and lift your head, then round your back like an angry cat and tuck your chin.

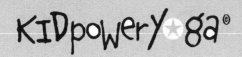

Butterfly (Video):
Sit on your bottom. Press the soles of the feet together with knees bent out to the sides. Place your hands on your shoulders to make wings or fingers to the head for antenna. Use your tongue as a proboscis to suck in nectar.

Ladybug (Video):
Come into a squat and bring your palms together in Namasté.

Spider:
Come into Ladybug and then place your hands on the floor for spider legs.

Happy Baby/Dead Bug:
Lie on your back and bend your knees. Grab the soles of your feet with your hands (or hold your shins). Let your spine sink into the floor and rock back and forth-side to side.

Boat (Video):
Sit on your bottom and balance as you lift your legs and hands off the floor.

Turtle (Video):
Start in Butterfly. Bring your legs out into a 'V' on the floor. Then bend your knees to the sides. Bring your palms to the floor between your legs and slide them under each arch of your knees. Tuck your head and then lift—repeat.

Cow:
Sit crisscrossed and then move one leg more or less over the top of the other. Knees are on top of one another. Feet are out to either side of the body.

Mermaid/Merman (Video):
Sit on your bottom and bring both legs bent and to one side (this is your tale). Bring your hand to your eyebrows and peer out—turning side to side to twist. Flip flap your tale to the other side and repeat.

Peacock:
This is a forward lunge. Come into Downward Dog and then bring the right foot forward between the hands (or as close as possible). Drop the back knee to the floor and lean forward into the lunge. If it is comfortable, bring your hands over your head.

Notes:

_____

_____

_____

_____

_____

_____

_____

_____

_____

_____

_____

_____

_____

_____

_____

_____

_____

_____

_____

_____

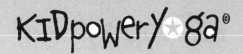

VIII. Vinyasa—Flows for Kids

Vinyasa: Sequencing Guidelines:

In creating vinyasa sequences for your classes, there are three guidelines to follow:

Move from Simple to Complex

Move from simple to complex movements, move from easy to hard. Generally, this translates to moving from the standing sequence to balancing postures to the floor, as you open the lines of the body. The idea is to go from stable (both feet on the floor) to unstable (one foot off the ground). It is not essential to get to complex or 'hard'. Each pose is a diagnostic tool, adding more complex postures only as needed. Some classes may not need them at all.

Try it Out

Try it out in your own body. Make sure that the movements and their sequence feel good to you. You should enjoy this flow as much as the students. When you are teaching a story driven flow, you may sacrifice some of the fluidity of your sequencing, but it should still feel good.

Stay in the Flow

Let your transitions be postures. As much as possible, allow students to stay in the flow by being as intentional as possible when moving from one posture to the next even when the transition is a bit choppy. (Exp. Being in a standing posture and needing to get to the floor without a very clear bridge between.)

Vinyasa: Flows for Kids

Good Night Yoga (Video)

The **sun** in the sky is **going down**
And the **clouds float by**
The **stars sparkle brightly**
As the **moon** rises high
The **birds** are heading back now
To their homes in the **trees**
The **ladybugs** have settled in for the night
Between the **butterflies** and the **bees**
And the little blue **cat** who lives in the moon whispers
"Good night world—You'll be dreaming soon."

Simple Flow (not story-based)

Simple Flow (Begin on your hands and knees/preparation for Cat Tilts)
Cat Tilts
Explorer Pose: On hands and knees: Right Arm Forward, Left Leg Extends Straight Back (balance).
Then switch sides: Left Arm Forward, Right Leg Extends Back (balance)

Note:

I have worked with classes of 10th graders who could not engage in the class if the flows were not story-based. I have also worked with Kindergarten classes who could actually do a 30 minute flow class that was as spontaneous as an adult class. Try not to presuppose what will work for your students, and when you find it—don't judge it. If they are doing yoga, that is success.

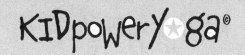

Upward Dog
Child Pose
(Repeat Upward Dog/Child Pose several times to warm up the spine)
Downward Dog
Half-Lunge (right foot forward)
Downward Dog
Half-Lunge (left foot forward)
Step Forward (both feet at the front of the mat)
Roll up to Standing Mountain Pose
Mountain Pose
Half-Moon (Standing) Both Sides
Star Pose
Horse
Ladybug
Seated Meditation Pose (criss-cross legs)

The Lonely Mountain (Video)

There once was a lonely mountain. (Mountain)
Streams rushed down her sides. (Arms and Hands awake)
Every once in a while beavers blocked the streams (Shoulders to Ears)
And then the water rushed through (3x) (Release)
Other than the beavers there were no friends on the mountain
One night there was a thunderstorm (Chair)
And lightening (Warrior II)
And then after a while the moon rose (Half Moon)
And out came the Stars (Star)
The mountain made a wish (Wish movement)
'I want friends on this mountain'
A magical volcano spirit heard the wish and filled the volcano with lava (Volcano)
The lava burst out over the mountain bringing new life (Erupt)
Monkeys came to the mountain (Gorilla)
Wild Horses came to the mountain (Horse)
Families of Ostriches came to the mountain (Ostrich)
Eagles flew over the mountain (Eagles)
And came to rest in its Trees (Tree)
Snakes came to play on the mountain (Cobra)
Wild Cats came to the mountain (Cat Tilts)
Prairie Dogs came to the mountain (Downward Dog-optional leg up for 'peeing')
Peacocks came proudly to the mountain (Peacock both sides)
Ladybugs came to the mountain (Ladybug)
Spiders came to the mountain

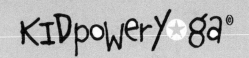

Butterflies came to the mountain (Butterfly)
Bees came to the mountain (Bee Breath)
And out on the rocks the Mermaids (Mermaid Twist)
And the Mermen (Merman Twist)
Watched the glorious celebration
On their Golden Rocks (Child Pose)
Rest

Make Your Own Vinyasa (Video)

There are many ways to do this. In the video, I had the students 'choose' the postures to be involved with their presentation, but they had been pre-selected so I did have control over what we were putting together.

You can:
- Create your own Vinyasa and teach it over time using the guidelines given here.
- Create your own Vinyasa with students in the moment (either with pre-selected poses or not. Without pre-selecting it is less clear what you'll end up with, but can still be a nice change of pace to try)
- Create a Vinyasa based on a story that you read as you go or reference throughout

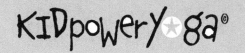

Notes:

_____

_____

_____

_____

_____

_____

_____

_____

_____

_____

_____

_____

_____

_____

_____

_____

_____

_____

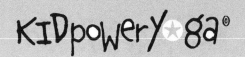

IX. Savasana

It is important to include some kind of relaxation (even 3 deep breaths) at the end of your classes. It is physically a way to let go of residual stress and re-integrate the movement that has happened in class. It is also a crucial teaching point; rest and relaxation are as essential as the movement. In a culture that prioritizes action, the power of inaction can't be taught enough.

How to Make it Work for Kids - Relaxation Tools

Keep it short until you can make it long:
A little goes a long way and don't be concerned with how much they do, just keep offering something. Many of them can access profound quiet in even an 8 count of meditation.

Use Tools:
Using tools such as squeezing and releasing—giving them something to 'do' while relaxing can be a way to get them moving in that direction.

Don't give up:
If you keep bringing them to a still place at the end of class, many of them will get there over time and often it becomes their favorite part.

Tensing and Relaxing:
Beginning with the face and shoulders, move up and down the body tensing and relaxing body parts.

Magic Carpet Ride/Guided Cloud Visualization - See Appendix

Meditation—8 Count: (Video)
Explain to the students that they will be doing a focused meditation using one of the 5 senses: Hearing. Guide them to become still and maybe even close their eyes or look down. Then you will lead them, speaking to an 8 count—reminding them to notice what they hear.

Color Visualization:
Have the students imagine that they are filling slowly with a calming color on an inhale (it can be helpful for you to give the guide like lavender or green) and then that they are exhaling all of the color back out. You can also use inhaling one color, and exhaling out another.

Notes:

_____

_____

_____

_____

_____

_____

_____

_____

_____

_____

_____

_____

_____

_____

_____

_____

_____

_____

_____

_____

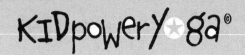

X. Breathing Techniques

As with the start of class, it is important to be intentional about your ending as well. This portion of class can also be limited by time constraints and it is wonderful to keep it very simple. The idea is to create the container for the experience of your students. We are always modeling for them and it continues right up to this point.

Ocean: (Video)
Very calming breath and is the young person's introduction to Ujay Breathing.

Bunny: (Video)
This is a wonderful 'wake up' breath. Recommendation: Do not use it more than 3xs/in a row before going back to normal breathing.

Bee: (Video)
Calming and fun.

Lion: (Video)
Great for getting out excess energy.

3–Part Breath: (Video)
Very calming and full body breath. Brings tactile awareness to the process of breath entering the body.

Filling Like a Balloon:
Similar to the 3 part breath, use the image of filling like a balloon to bring students' attention to taking in full breaths.

Balloon Breath:
This can be done by taping a balloon to each students torso or using small stuffed animals. Once the object is in place, have the students breathe fully so they can watch the rise and fall of the object. Increases awareness of full breathing.

Cotton Ball/Straw:
Have each student at one end of the room with a cotton ball and a straw. Have them use their breath only to propel the cotton ball to the other side of the room. Increases awareness of breathing.

Notes:

_____

_____

_____

_____

_____

_____

_____

_____

_____

_____

_____

_____

_____

_____

_____

_____

_____

_____

_____

_____

_____

_____

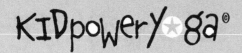

XI. Closing Rituals

As with the start of class, it is important to be intentional about your ending as well. This portion of class can also be limited by time constraints and it is wonderful to keep it very simple. The idea is to create the container for the experience of your students. We are always modeling for them and it continues right up to this point.

A Closing Ritual may be:
Namasté (Video) hands in prayer at the chest—Meaning: 'The Light in me sees the Light in you' at the end of the class to each other and to oneself (acknowledging our own light).

★ Silent Applause (Video): The sign language of shaking hands in the air

★ Silent Cheer (Video): A wild raucous cheer—with no sound.

★ Spraying down or rolling up of the mats: It may be that the real closure comes with the clear process of literally respectfully finishing the use of the space.

It does not matter what it is, it matters that you have some intention behind it.

Notes:

_____

_____

_____

_____

_____

_____

_____

_____

_____

_____

_____

_____

_____

_____

_____

_____

_____

_____

_____

_____

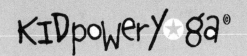

MORE TOOLS

XII. Pre-K through High School; Working with different ages

This program and model are used for pre-K students all the way through high school. Modifications should be made, but the overall structure and approach are the same.

Do not be afraid to use the more playful warm ups to bring a group of older students into the practice. They need the ease and light-heartedness, the play, as much as the 2nd graders if not more. When I teach a warm up like 'Tippy Toes' or 'Sometimes' with older students, it is my presentation that changes. I teach it to them with a bit of a 'wink' as in: 'We both know this a little silly… let's get moving!' If students are laughing, but actually doing the exercise; that is success.

I have worked with groups of 10th graders who could not stay connected to a flow class unless it was strongly story based. In contrast, I've also worked with kindergartners who could easily follow a flow class. Don't make assumptions about an age group or judge the response, just respond to your students so they can be successful.

Of course, there are groups of older students who can participate in an essentially adult yoga class. If you have a group of students who are capable in this way, adjust the structure in the following manner:

Class Elements: Advanced Groups

Optional: (Ritual) This would be, as in an adult class, removing shoes, laying out one's mat, getting props if needed.

I. Warm Up:
This could be the start of the class—Sun Salutations A + Sun Salutations B (see appendix)

II. Building Blocks:
If needed, you could workshop 1-2 poses or particular alignment points to be incorporated into the flow as a quick pause or at the very start of the session.

III. Vinyasa:
A flowing class using the Kid Power Yoga flows without the narrative or creating your own using the sequencing techniques.

IV. Savasana/Relaxation:
Savasana

V. Closing Ritual:

Coming up to a seated position—Namasté—hands in prayer and a bow.

44

Poses

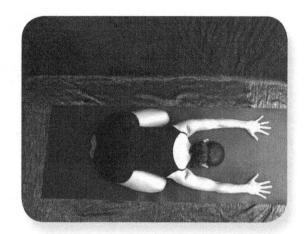

Childs Pose

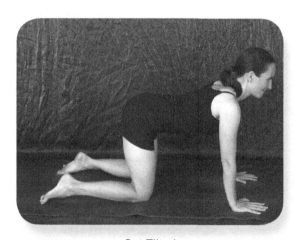

Cat Tilts I

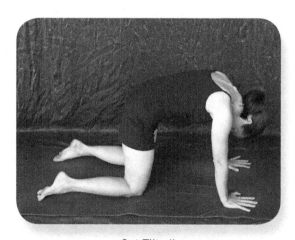

Cat Tilts II

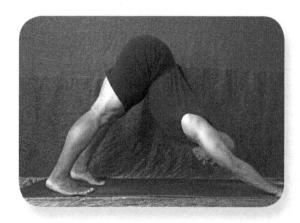

Downward Dog

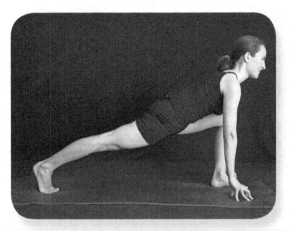

Lunge Left

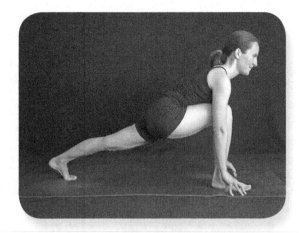

Lunge Right

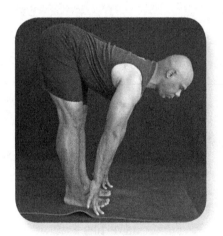

Extension

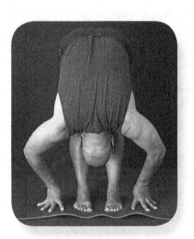

Fold Forward

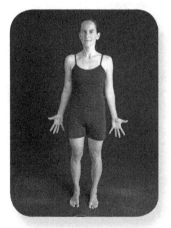

Mountain

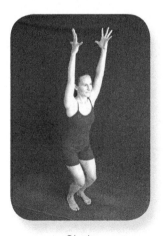

Chair

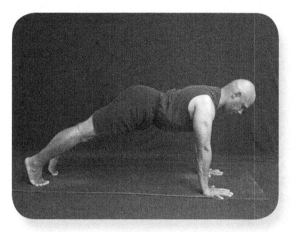

Plank

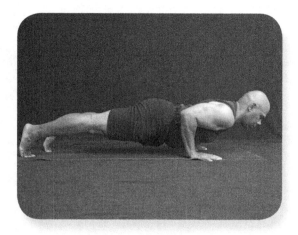

Low Plank

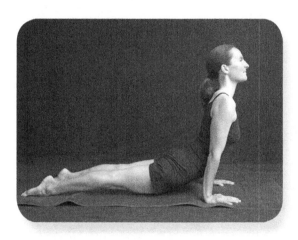

Upward Dog

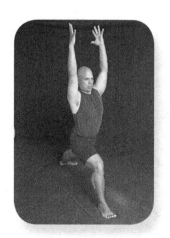

Warrior I

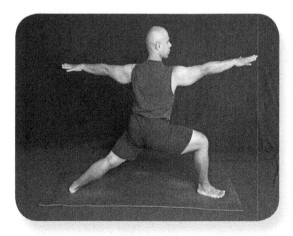

Warrior II

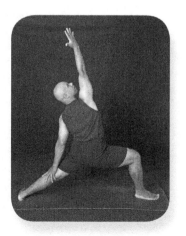

Reverse Warrior

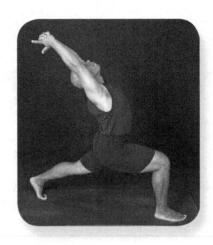

Warrior Lunge

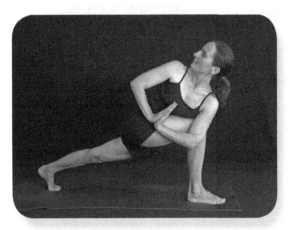

Twisting Lunge I

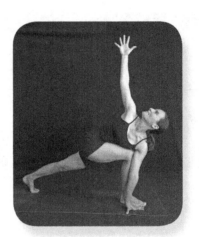

Twisting Lunge II

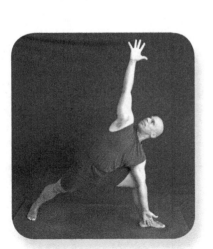

Bent Knee Triangle

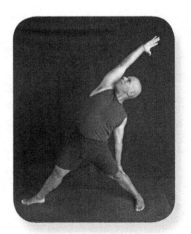

Reverse Triangle

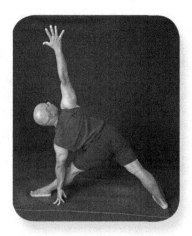

Triangle

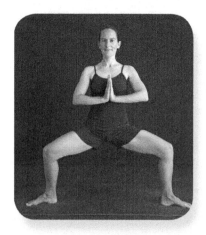

Horse

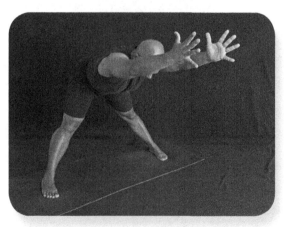

Core Line Extension

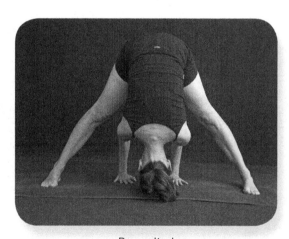

Prasarita I

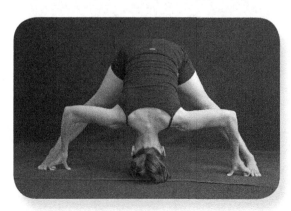

Prasarita II

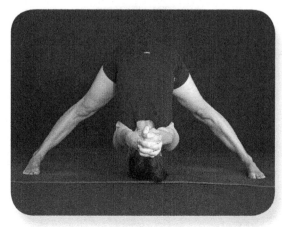

Prasarita III

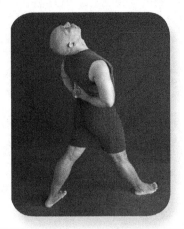

Parsvottanasana I

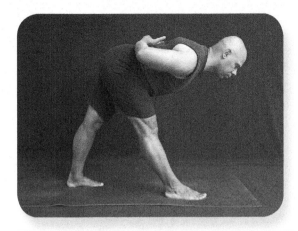

Parsvottanasana II

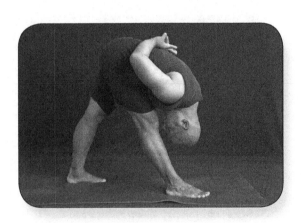

Parsvottanasana III

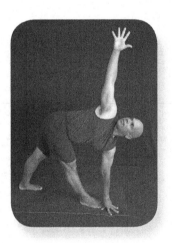

Twisting Triangle

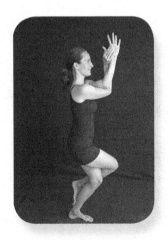

Eagle

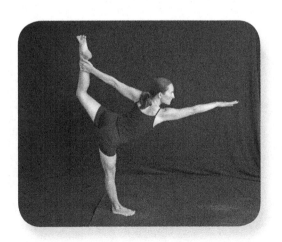

Dancer

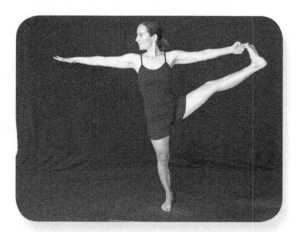

Hand to Foot Extension

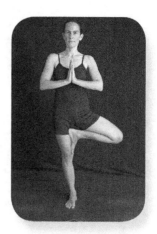

Tree

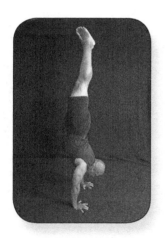

Handstand

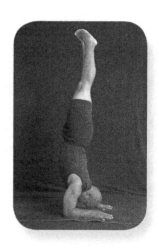

Forearm Stand

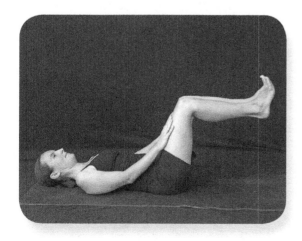

Core Work I

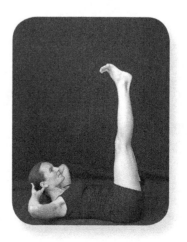

Core Work II

KIDpowerYoga©

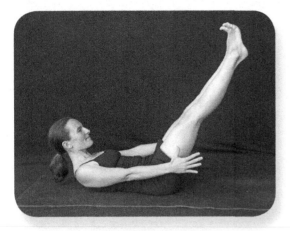

Core Work III

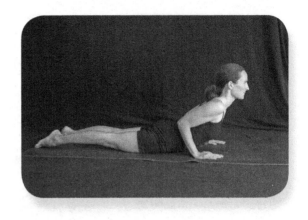

Cobra

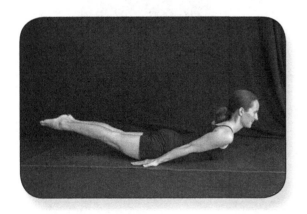

Locust

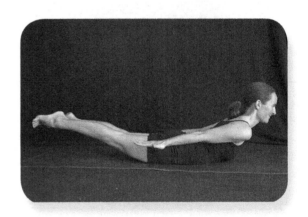

Bow I

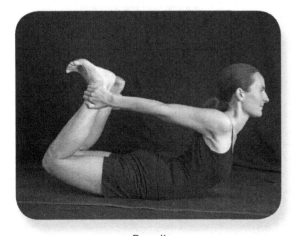

Bow II

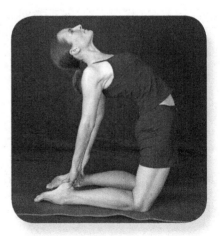

Camel

52

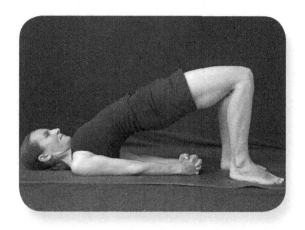

Bridge

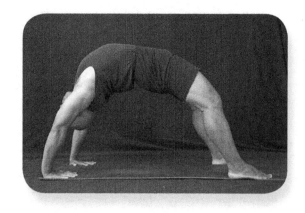

Wheel

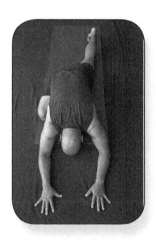

Pigeon

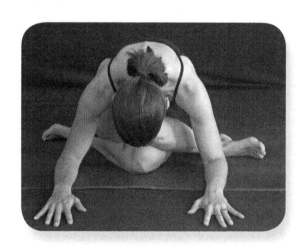

Cow Face

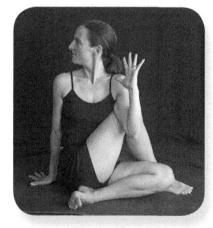

Seated Twist

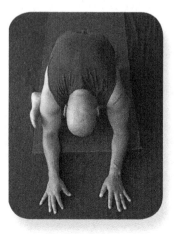

Double Pigeon

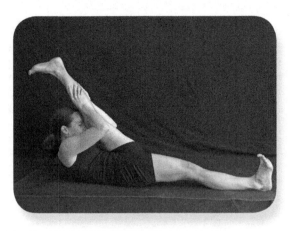

Reclining Forehead to Knee

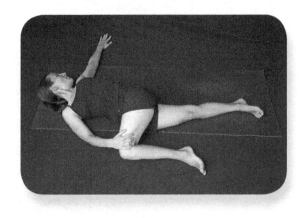

Knee Down Twist

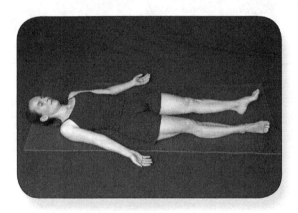

Savasana

Sun Salutation A

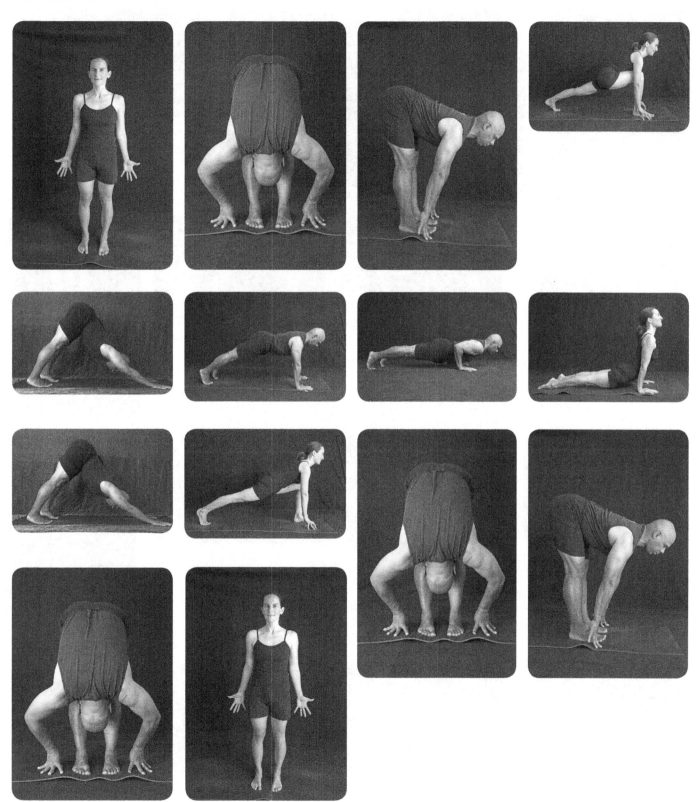

Sun Salutation B

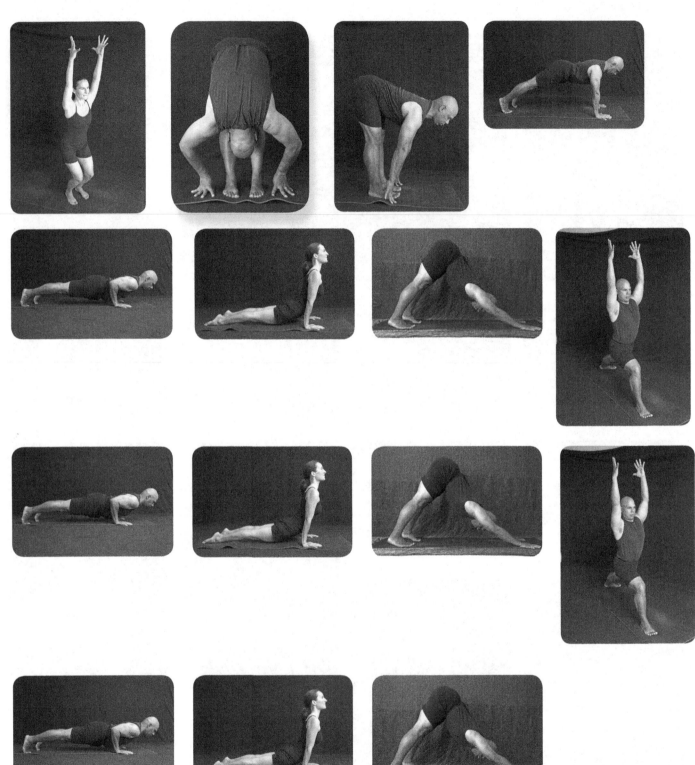

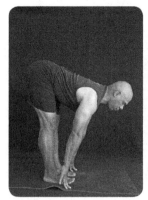 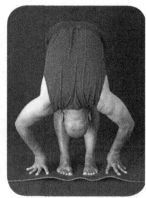 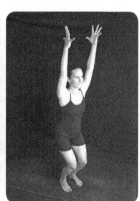

KIDpowerYoga®

The Good Night Yoga Flow
From *Good Night Yoga: A Pose by Pose Bedtime Story* by Mariam Gates

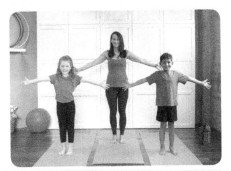
Sun Breath

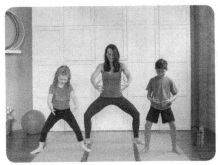
Cloud Gathering

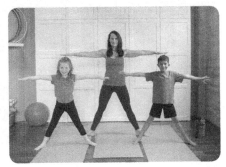
Star

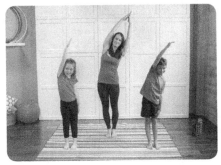
Half Moon

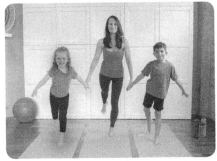
Bird

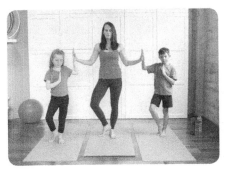
Tree

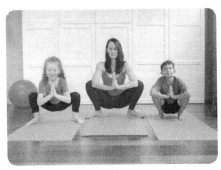
Ladybug

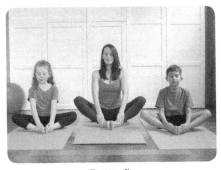
Butterfly

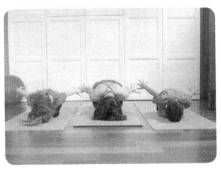
Bee

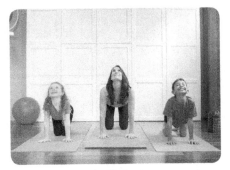
Cat

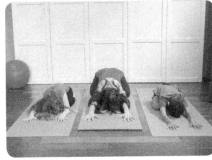
Child Pose

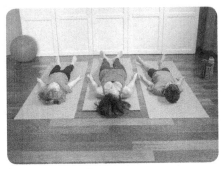
Savasana

58

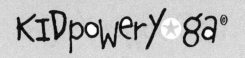

Notes:

_____

_____

_____

_____

_____

_____

_____

_____

_____

_____

_____

_____

_____

_____

_____

_____

_____

_____

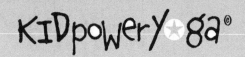

XIII. The Yamas and Niyamas with Young People

The Yamas (The Restraints) and Niyamas (Observances) represent the basic do's and don'ts of the Eight Limb Path and yoga's approach to a sustainable life.

The Eight-Limb Path of Yoga

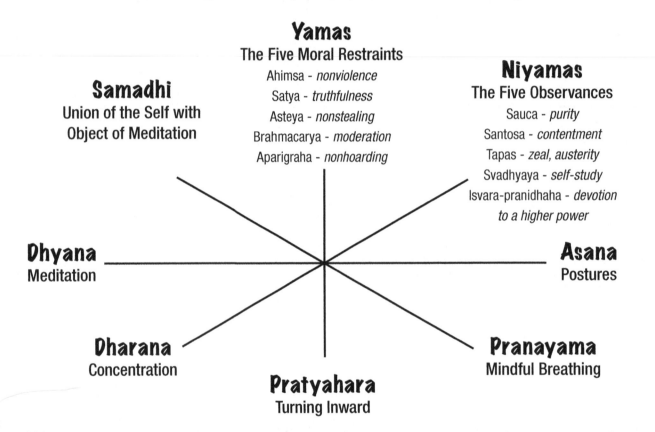

The Two Aspects of Spiritual Practice

Abhyasa - *practice*
Vairagya - *renunciation*

The Four Aims of Life

Dharma - *observation of spiritual discipline*
Artha - *creation of a balanced life*
Kama - *enjoyment of the fruits of one's labors*
Moksa - *liberation*

The Five Afflictions

Avidya - *spiritual ignorance*
Asmita - *pride*
Raga - *desire*
Dvesa - *aversion*
Abhinivesa - *fear of death*

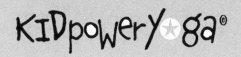

Ahimsa: Non-violence	Satya: Truthfulness	Asetya: Non-stealing	Brahmacarya: Moderation	Aparigraha: Non-hoarding

Yamas: The Five Moral Restraints

Sauca: Purity	Santosa: Contentment	Tapas: Zeal	Svadhyaya: Self-Study	Isvara-pranidhana: Devotion to a Higher Power

Niyamas: The Five Observances

There are different ways to approach yogic philosophy with young people. As you can see, the guidelines here are not much different from the basic beliefs of a functioning society (even when we may not always practice them). Trust that by teaching thoroughly and with emphasis, the essence of yoga is being conveyed along with the actual poses i.e., the Truthfulness and Nonviolence of being gentle with yourself in a pose, the Purity of placing your shoes and yoga mat, the Zeal brought to a practice, and the Moderation used when going into a posture, such as Airplane pose.

It can also be fun to do some specific work around these teachings:

If you have the ability to take students outside, a powerful exercise can be to go on a walk with the awareness of Ahimsa/nonviolence and Asetya/non-stealing. Non-violence as you walk, and also non-stealing, not taking things that are not ours to take (a leaf off of a tree, a spider's careful web)—really noticing what kind of an effect we have sometimes without even seeing it.

With older students, the teachings can evolve to other levels:

★ Pick one chore the student does not like to do, such as; laundry, math homework, or taking out the trash. Ask them to experiment with doing that chore with Tapas/Zeal. What does it feel like to fully bring yourself into an activity—even if it is not your favorite task? Ask if using a different approach changes the experience and have them write about it.

★ Try practicing contentment for 15 minutes on the clock, or for 5 minutes within the class. Experiment with the feeling of contentment by using a clear memory and image of when everything felt alright, and then have students work on staying with that feeling for 5 minutes while the class continues. Debrief at the end, sharing what was or was not challenging about the exercise. Also, engage in a discussion of why cultivating a feeling of contentment would be a worthwhile practice in life. Why is it one of the Niyamas?

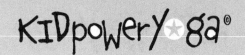

XIV. Strategies for School Programs

How to Approach:
Teaching in schools is very exciting because in many cases, this will be students' first exposure to yoga. It is ideal to have a connection to the school you wish to teach in, but it is not essential. Making a request to speak with the principal, guidance counselor or PTA members will get you in front of the decision-makers.

How to Schedule:
Most schools love the idea of bringing in a yoga class in the following ways:

- As a classroom mini-break in the day.
- As a replacement for Gym (many schools no longer offer a dedicated gym class).
- As a before or after-school program.
- As a paid after-school class (many schools offer after-school self-development classes, such as dance or chess).

If you are trying a new venue, it makes sense to begin with a 6-10 week program and then assess the viability and/or need for adjustments.

How to Fund:*
There are so many ways to find funding for teaching in schools. There are many websites offering funding for programs and Kid Power Yoga can offer additional support around grant writing if you are newer to the work.

Faster ways to find funding include:

- Principal funding the class
- PTA funding the class (Parent organizations fund raise to bring in outside resources the schools would otherwise be without. In some cases they may be willing to also be involved in grant writing).
- Students pay individually for an after school program

Some grants require assessment (an evaluation of the students before and after your course. This is much simpler to accomplish than it sounds and the Kid Power Yoga office can help you navigate assessment tools if needed.

*If you are agreeing to volunteer as a yoga teacher because you want the practice and are excited by working in schools, again be sure to have clear agreements in place around the length of your teaching commitment so you can then assess your next steps.

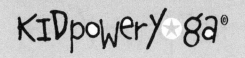

Notes:

_____

_____

_____

_____

_____

_____

_____

_____

_____

_____

_____

_____

_____

_____

_____

_____

_____

_____

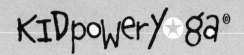

XV. Strategies for Studios and for Community Center Programs

How to Approach:
Studios - If you love your studio and they do not currently offer kids' yoga or only offer it at specific times/age groups, submit your resume and ask to start a new class. You may want to offer to guest teach or offer a one time special class at the location.

Community Centers - Most communities are usually looking for new offerings. Check out the local recreation center/adult education programming and submit a proposal. One added benefit with a recreation center is that it will handle the registrations.

How to Schedule:
Studio + Community Center Classes: Instructors must schedule classes so the kids can attend.
For younger classes and Parent + Me (under 5) mornings are fine.

For all other classes: Afternoons

    5-7 years: 45 minutes - 1hr (45 minutes is best, but tight for parents dropping off and picking up.)
    8-11 years: 1hr
    12-14 years: 1hr

How to Fund:
Studio + Community Center Classes - A studio or recreation center will take a percentage of class revenue. The amount will vary from place to place. If you are renting a space and marketing your own class, you may find a better financial arrangement, but then you sacrifice the exposure of a larger, more established location. This is a matter of choice, both strategies can be successful.

When setting fees, take the following into account;

• Estimate expenses such as props, supplies, etc.

• Research fees at other yoga studios and be competitive. The range falls between $8-$15 per class, with a discount for paying in full.

Series vs. Drop In:
This is again, a personal choice. Overall, I offer courses as a set series of classes that are paid for whether or not the student attends. I want to establish consistency for myself and the students and this makes the commitment very clear.

I also offer the 'drop in class' at a slightly higher rate because I find it is necessary to attract new students and their families and introduce them to my classes.

Notes:

_____

_____

_____

_____

_____

_____

_____

_____

_____

_____

_____

_____

_____

_____

_____

_____

_____

_____

_____

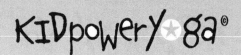

XVI. Appendix:

Mind Mapping: Examples

Mind Mapping: Templates

KPY Class: Examples

KPY Class: Templates

The 5 Core Principles of Teaching: Class Assessment

The 5 Core Principles of Teaching: Self-Assessment

Terms Glossary

Advanced Flow: Sun Salutation (A + B)

Parent Contact Information-Sample

Parent Waiver-Sample

Parent Photo Release-Sample

Narrative Class Cards

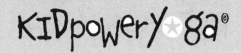

Mind Mapping: Samples

Use the middle point and then connect the comments around like mind mapping/brainstorming.

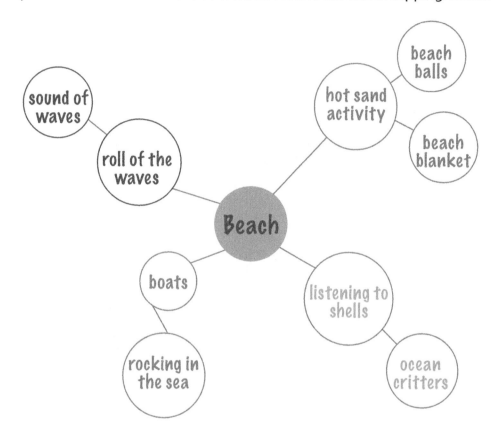

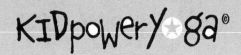

Mind Mapping: Samples

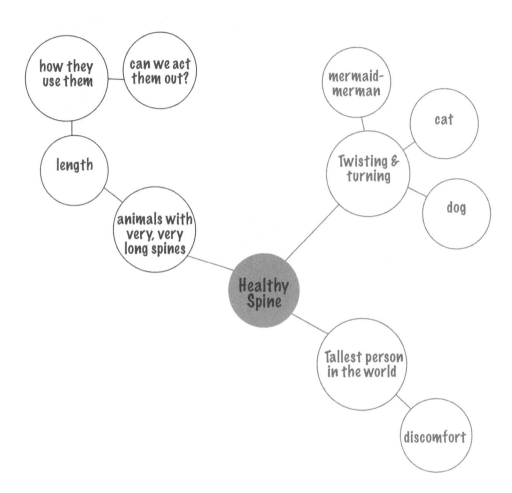

Mind Mapping: Samples

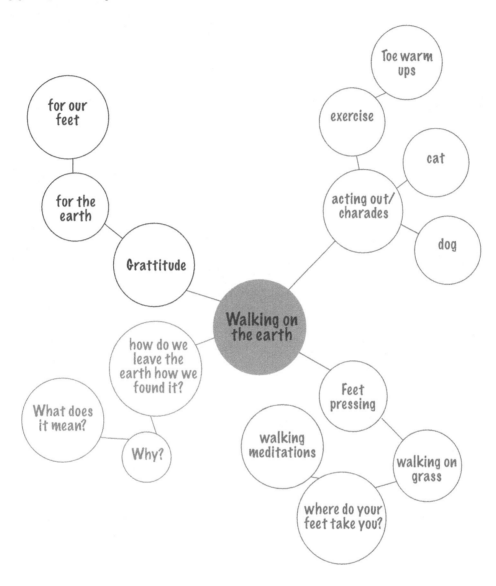

Central: **Walking on the earth**

- **Grattitude**
  - for the earth
    - for our feet
- **acting out/ charades**
  - exercise
    - Toe warm ups
  - cat
  - dog
- **how do we leave the earth how we found it?**
  - What does it mean?
  - Why?
- **Feet pressing**
  - walking meditations
  - where do your feet take you?
  - walking on grass

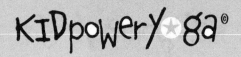

Mind Mapping

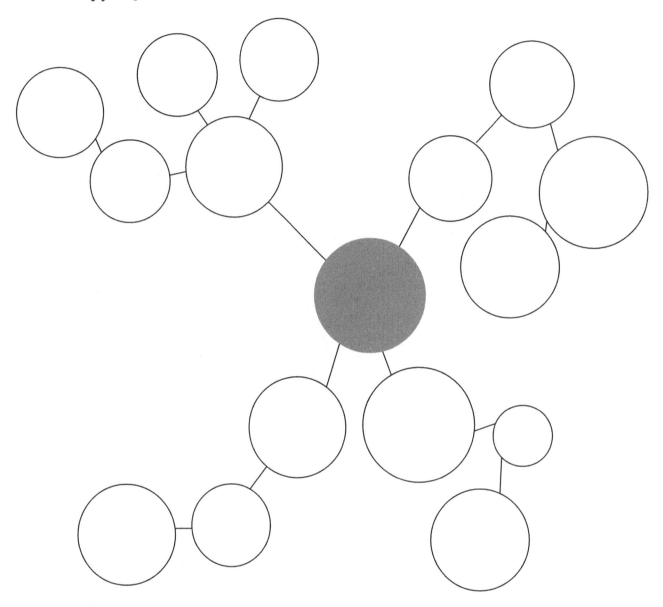

Mind Mapping

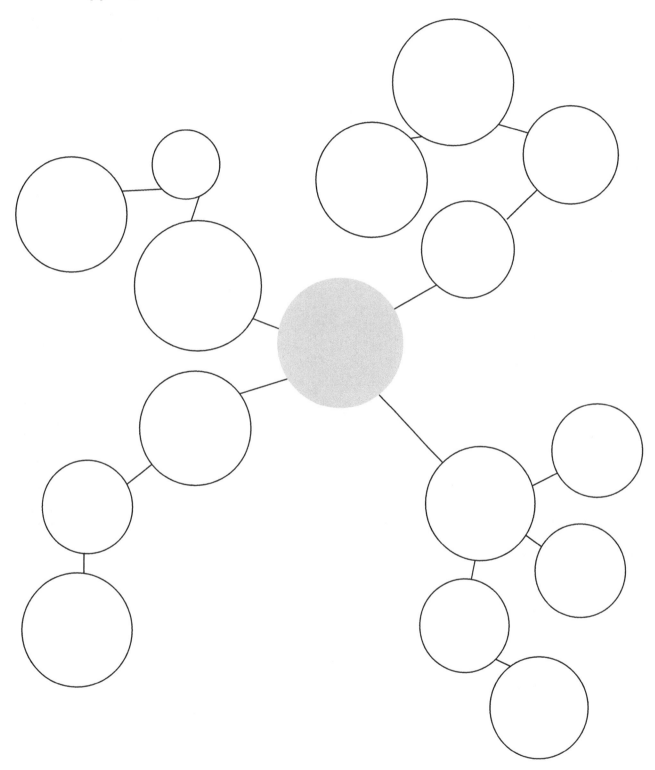

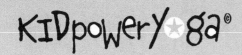

Mind Mapping

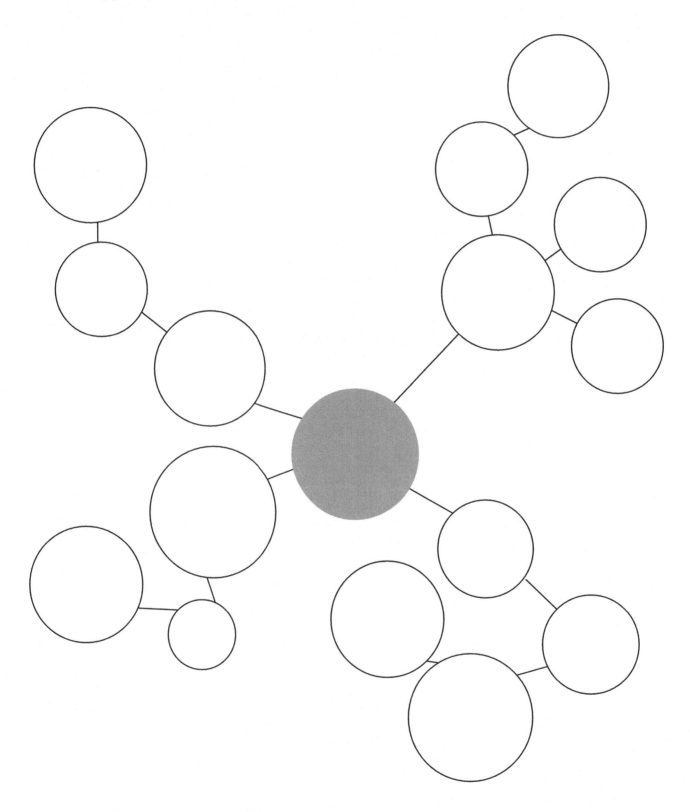

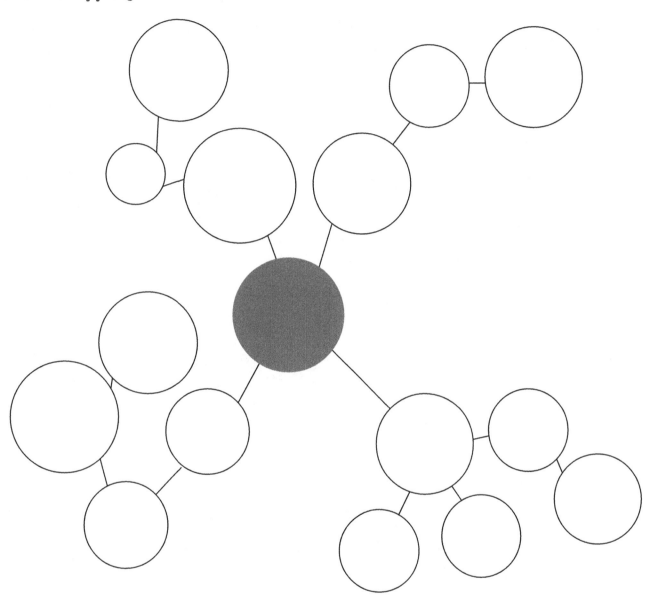

Mind Mapping

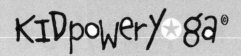

Mind Mapping

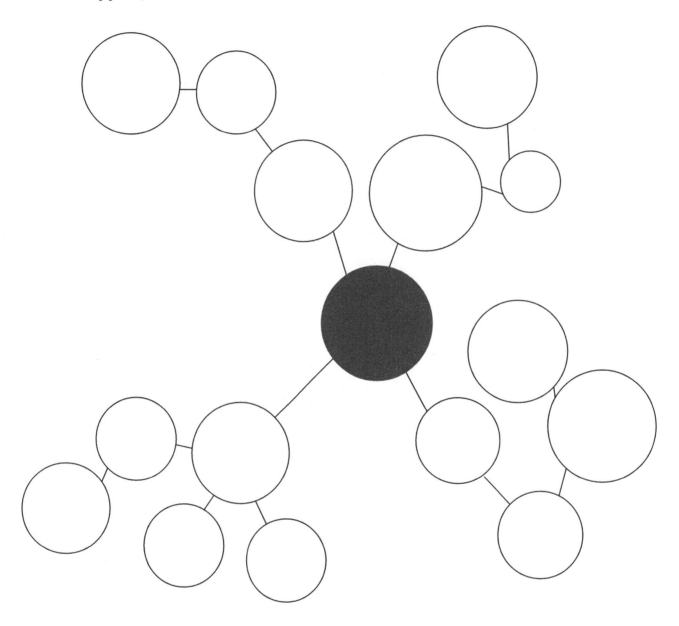

74

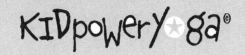

KPY Class: Examples

Class Theme: My Spine is Fine
Length of Class: 1hr
Location: Studio
Ritual: Removing Shoes
Warm Ups: Cat Tilts/Side movements/Cobra/Child pose flow/Pipe Cleaners
Building Blocks: Follow Me: Cat/Dog/Tree/Mermaid
Vinyasa: The Lonely Mountain
Savasana: Belly Breathing
Closing Ritual
Silent Cheer
Namasté

What will you bring in if you have extra time?
Expand on balloon breathing--3 part belly breathing before savasana if time

Any props needed: (music, your notes, physical props etc.)
Pipe Cleaners
Music for warm up and vinyasa

Class Theme: Walking on the Earth
Length of Class: 1hr
Location: Studio
Ritual: Art activity: Tracing our feet and drawing somewhere we love to go inside the foot
Warm Up: Toe Warm Up/Massage + Tippy Toes
Building Blocks: Workshop: 1/2 moon, tree, bird
Vinyasa: Good Night Yoga
Savasana: Tense and Relax
Closing Ritual
Fingertips touching—exhale Peeeeaaaaccccceeee for the earth (3xs)
Namasté

Class Theme: A Day at the Beach
Length of Class: 40 minutes
Location: Classroom
Ritual: Taking off shoes—putting carefully out of the way
Warm Ups: Beach Ball Toss/Team Building
Building Blocks: Postures out of the net (Feet/Hands/Eyes)-emphasis
Vinyasa: Turtle Story
Savasana: Cloud Visualization
Closing Ritual: Silent Cheer
Namasté

What will you bring in if you have extra time?
8 count meditation

Any props needed: (music, your notes, physical props, etc.)
Beach Ball
Net
Toys/postures in net
Waves or whales sound track—music

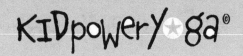

Building a Class: Template

Class Theme -

Length of Class -

Location -

Ritual -

Warm Ups -

Building Blocks -

Vinyasa -

Savasana -

Closing Ritual -

What will you bring in if you have extra time? -

Any props needed - (music, your notes, physical props etc.)

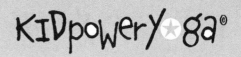

The Magic Carpet Ride - A Guided Meditation.

Also see *Good Night Yoga: A Pose by Pose Bedtime Story* **by Mariam Gates for a** *Cloud Journey Visualization*

"Let your body become quiet and still on the mat and if you want to—try closing your eyes even just a bit. Imagine now that your mat has become a magic carpet beneath you. Slowly feel as you begin to rise up from the floor on your carpet as it takes you gently and safely into the air.

Your carpet brings you slowly out the door and onto the street where you fly up over the buildings. See if you can feel the gentle rocking it gives you as you sail out over the city and over fields and valleys below. Feel yourself flying over an ocean all the way to a beautiful mountain.

As you come closer to the mountain, you see that there is a beautiful waterfall rushing down the side—glistening in the sun. The carpet brings you closer and you can feel how warm and inviting the water is. You move closer and feel the warm light water rushing down over your head, and down your shoulders, your arms, your body. The water is sparkling and light and keeps pouring over you making you feel very, very relaxed.

You realize then that it is time to go back and the carpet slowly pulls away from the waterfall—you thank the waterfall as you move away back over the ocean, back over the fields and valleys, back over the city. And then you are just over this studio—and magically, the carpet comes back through the door and all the way into this room. Then it settles you all the way back down to the floor.

Feel how your body is touching the floor now and how the solid earth is supporting your body as it lays on the floor."

Continuation: Releasing of Worry

"And notice, that something is floating up and out of you and away. It is blue and purple and swirling and is all of your worries, all of your concerns, anything that is bothering you. You are so relaxed that it is all floating up and back to the universe and you do not have to worry—everything will be taken care of.

On the day you were born, a miracle happened—you came into the world because the world needed someone exactly like you. So all you have to do now is be exactly you—all you have to do is be…
Alex… India… Colin… and the universe will take care of everything else… that is all you have to do…
Now roll slowly onto your right side…"

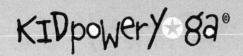

The 5 Core Principles of Teaching: Class Assessment

Class Assessment & Discussion Points

1. Preparation
What kind of preparation was needed for this class? How were the kids prepared when moving into each segment of the class? How would you have prepared for this class?

2. Connection
Where did you see examples of connection? What was working?

3 Tempo
What did you notice about the tempo of the class? How were the transitions?

4. Emphasis
What supported the emphasis of the class? How was the emphasis made clear?

5. Self Study

Where would this curriculum have pushed you? What do you want to know more about?

The 5 Core Principles of Teaching: Self-Assessment

SELF ASSESSMENT
What do I notice about this principle in my teaching?

How do I feel about my_____?

1. Preparation

2. Connection

3. Tempo

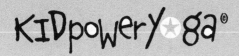

4. Emphasis

5. Self Study

Poses

Sun Salutation A

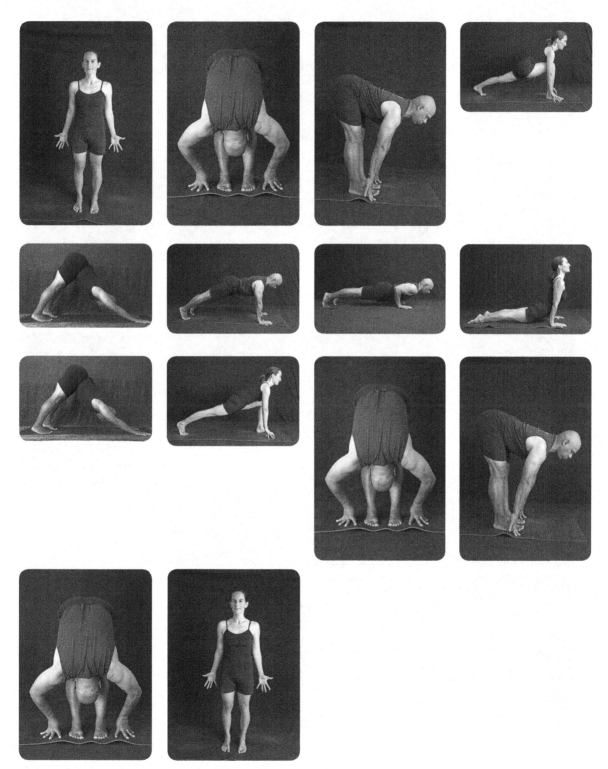

KIDpowerY★ga©

Sun Salutation B

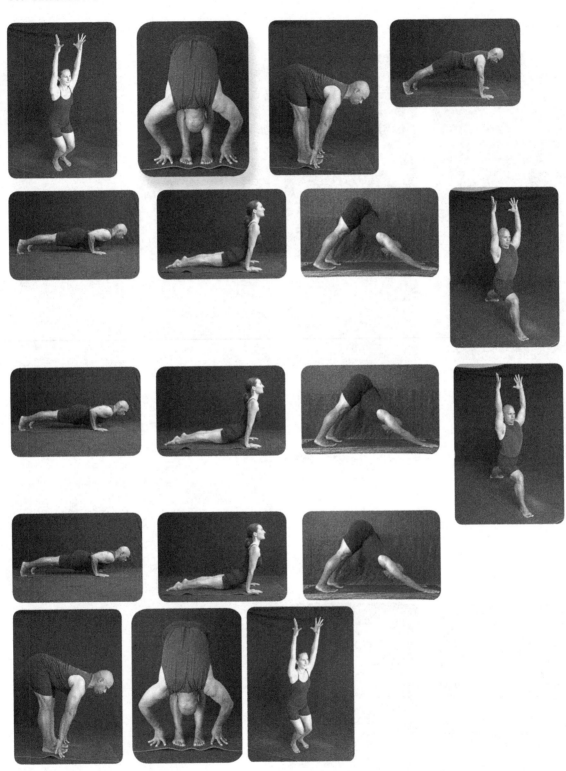

Parent Contact Information - Sample

Student Name: _____

Parent/s Name: _____

Address: _____

Email: _____

Phone Number/s: _____

Emergency Contact: _____

1. Is there anyone beside yourself who is authorized to pick your child/children up from Kid Power Yoga? (Please also list spouse/parent).

_____

2. Is there anything you would like us to know about your child emotionally or physically? (Please also include any allergies or medical conditions/concerns)

_____

_____

3. Finally, what do you hope your child/children will get out of his/her Kid Power Yoga experience?

_____

_____

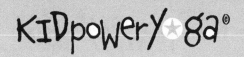

Agreement of Release and Waiver of Liability

(Please consult your own legal advice when designing your waivers. This is meant as a sample only.)

I agree to the following:

- I hereby authorize my child/children to participate in the Kid Power Yoga class (under the supervision of_____ being offered at the _____STUDIO (Physical Address) during which he/she/ they will receive information and instruction on yoga, movement and health.

- I recognize that yoga requires physical exertion, which may be strenuous and may cause physical injury and I am fully aware of the risks and hazards involved. In consideration of this, I agree to assume full responsibility for any risks, injuries or damages, known or unknown, which my child or children might incur as a result of participating in the class. I represent and warrant that my child/children are physically fit and have no medical conditions which would prevent their full participation in Kid Power Yoga classes

- I knowingly, voluntarily and expressly waive any claim I or my child/children may have against Kid Power Yoga or Mariam Gates, or STUDIO for any injury or damages that they may sustain as a result of participating in the Kid Power Yoga program.

I have read the above release and waiver of liability, fully understand its contents and voluntarily agree to the terms and conditions stated above.

Signed: _____   Date: _____

Print: _____

Child's Name: _____

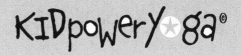

PHOTOS Waiver - Sample

Dear Kid Power Yoga Families,

From time to time we will take photos of the Kid Power Yoga classes that we plan to use for fliers and website information. Please sign this following permission form if you are willing to allow us to use pictures featuring your amazing KPY kids for these purposes.

Thank you for your help and for having such great kids!

I _____ give my permission to have photos featuring my

child/children _____ shown in promotional materials for Kid Power Yoga.

No, please do not use any pictures/video clips of my child _____

Signed _____ Date _____

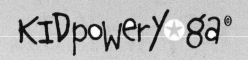

Notes:

KPY Yoga Class - Walking on the Earth

Warm Up: Waking up the
Feet +Tippy Toes

Building Blocks: Postures with
the emphasis on feet

Vinyasa: Good Night Yoga
(feel your feet pressing into the earth)

Savasana Relaxation—tense and
release—gratitude

KPY Yoga Class - Day at the Beach

Warm Up: Beach Ball passing with
music or parachute/picinic with
sea creatures

Building blocks: Pulling poses out
of a net to introduce
Vinyasa: Create your own flow based on
the ocean
(Turtle story)

Savasana: Cloud Visualization

KPY Yoga Class - My Spine is Fine

Warm Up: Pipe Cleaners + tactile

Building Blocks: Pick postures that
emphasize spine

Movement: Cat Tilts, Half Moon, Bird,
Mermaid/Merman

(Let's feel our spine here… and here…)

Vinyasa: The Lonely Mountain

Savasana: Filling Like a Balloon
getting long

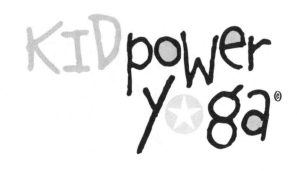

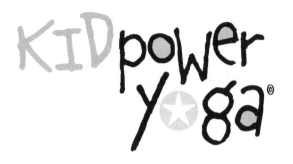

Good Night Yoga

The sun in the sky is going down

And the clouds float by

The stars sparkle brightly

As the moon rises high

The birds are heading back now

To their homes in the trees

The ladybugs have settled in for the night

Between the butterflies and the bees

And the little blue cat who lives
in the moon whispers

"Good night world—You'll be dreaming soon."

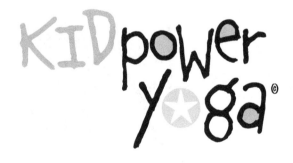

Lonely Mountain
There once was a lonely mountain. (Mountain)
Streams rushed down her sides. (Arms and Hands awake)
Every once in a while beavers blocked the streams (Shoulders to Ears)
And then the water rushed through (3x) (Release)
Other than the beavers there were no friends on the mountain
One night there was a thunderstorm (Chair)
And lightening (Warrior II)
And then after a while the moon rose (Half Moon)
And out came the Stars (Star)
The mountain made a wish (Wish movement)
'I want friends on this mountain'
A magical volcano spirit heard the wish and filled the volcano with lava (Volcano)
The lava burst out over the mountain bringing new life (Erupt)
Monkeys came to the mountain (Gorilla)
Snakes came to play on the mountain (Cobra)
Wild Cats came to the mountain (Cat Tilts)
Prairie Dogs came to the mountain (Downward Dog-optional leg up for 'peeing')
Peacocks came proudly to the mountain (Peacock both sides)
Ladybugs came to the mountain (Ladybug)
Spiders came to the mountain
Butterflies came to the mountain (Butterfly)
Bees came to the mountain (Bee Breath)
And out on the rocks the Mermaids (Mermaid Twist)
And the Mermen (Merman Twist)
Watched the glorious celebration
On their Golden Rocks (Child Pose)
Rest

Made in the
USA
Monee, IL